EASY KETO DIET RECIPES 2021

MOUTH-WATERING RECIPES EASY TO MAKE FOR BEGINNERS

TONY KEY

Table of Contents

Introduction 6
   Amazing Halibut Soup 11
   Simple Kimchi 13
   Delicious Green Beans Side Dish 15
   Simple Cauliflower Mash 17
   Delicious Portobello Mushrooms 19
   Brussels Sprouts Side Dish 21
   Delicious Pesto 23
   Brussels Sprouts And Bacon 25
   Delicious Spinach Side Dish 27
   Amazing Avocado Fries 30
   Simple Roasted Cauliflower 32
   Mushroom And Spinach Side Dish 34
   Delicious Okra And Tomatoes 36
   Amazing Snap Peas And Mint 38
   Collard Greens Side Dish 40
   Eggplant And Tomato Side Dish 42
   Broccoli With Lemon Almond Butter 44
   Delicious Pesto Crackers 46
   Pumpkin Muffins 48
   Delicious Bombs 50
   Special Tortilla Chips 53
   Amazing Jalapeno Balls 55
   Cheeseburger Muffins 57
   Tasty Pizza Dip 59
   Incredible Keto Muffins Snack 61
   Amazing Fried Queso Snack 64
   Maple And Pecan Bars 66
   Summer Side Salad 68
   Tomato And Bocconcini 70
   Cucumber And Dates Salad 72
   Easy Eggplant Salad 74
   Special Side Salad 76
   Special Endives And Watercress Side Salad 78

- Indian Side Salad 80
- Indian Mint Chutney 82
- Indian Coconut Chutney 84
- Easy Tamarind Chutney 86
- Caramelized Bell Peppers 88
- Caramelized Red Chard 91

Conclusion 94
- Avocado Dip 95
- Special Prosciutto And Shrimp Appetizer 97
- Broccoli And Cheddar Biscuits 100
- Tasty Corndogs 102
- Tasty Pepper Nachos 104
- Almond Butter Bars 106

Conclusion 108

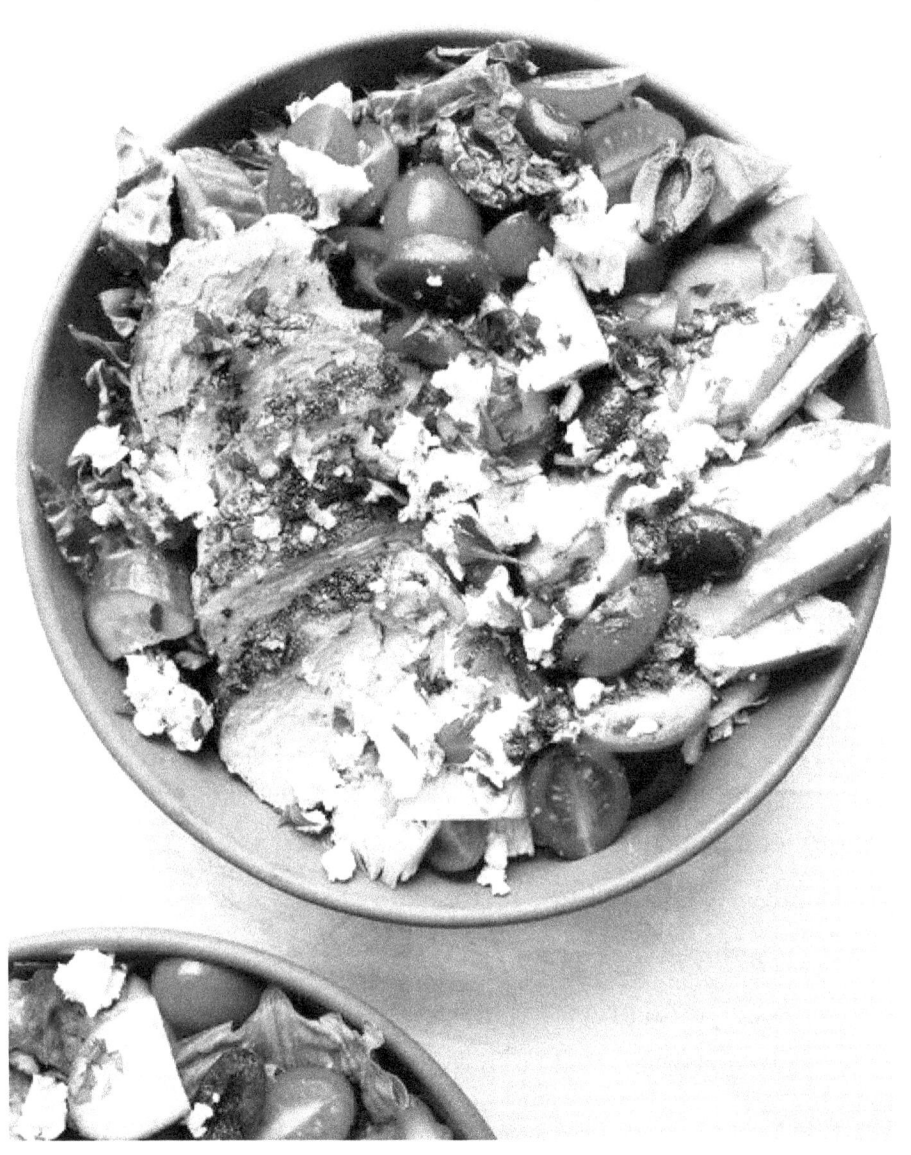

Introduction

Do you want to make a change in your life? Do you want to become a healthier person who can enjoy a new and improved life? Then, you are definitely in the right place. You are about to discover a wonderful and very healthy diet that has changed millions of lives. We are talking about the Ketogenic diet, a lifestyle that will mesmerize you and that will make you a new person in no time. So, let's sit back, relax and find out more about the Ketogenic diet.

A keto diet is a low carb one. This is the first and one of the most important things you should now. During such a diet, your body makes ketones in your liver and these are used as energy.
Your body will produce less insulin and glucose and a state of ketosis is induced.
Ketosis is a natural process that appears when our food intake is lower than usual. The body will soon adapt to this state and therefore you will be able to lose weight in no time but you will also become healthier and your physical and mental performances will improve.
Your blood sugar levels will improve and you won't be predisposed to diabetes.

Also, epilepsy and heart diseases can be prevented if you are on a Ketogenic diet.

Your cholesterol will improve and you will feel amazing in no time. How does that sound?

A Ketogenic diet is simple and easy to follow as long as you follow some simple rules. You don't need to make huge changes but there are some things you should know.

So, here goes!

If you are on a Ketogenic diet you can't eat:
- Grains like corn, cereals, rice, etc
- Fruits like bananas
- Sugar
- Dry beans
- Honey
- Potatoes
- Yams

If you are on a Ketogenic diet you can eat:
- Greens like spinach, green beans, kale, bok choy, etc
- Meat like poultry, fish, pork, lamb, beef, etc
- Eggs
- Above ground veggies like cauliflower or broccoli, napa cabbage or regular cabbage
- Nuts and seeds
- Cheese
- Ghee or butter
- Avocados and all kind of berries
- Sweeteners like erythritol, splenda, stevia and others that contain only a few carbs
- Coconut oil
- Avocado oil
- Olive oil

The list of foods you are allowed to eat during a keto diet is permissive and rich as you can see for yourself.
So, we think it should be pretty easy for you to start such a diet.

If you've made this choice already, then, it's time you checked our amazing keto recipe collection.

In this guide you will discover 50 of the best Ketogenic recipes for your lunch in the world and you will soon be able to make each and every one of these recipes.

Now let's start our magical culinary journey!
Ketogenic lifestyle...here we come!
Enjoy!

Amazing Halibut Soup

If you are following a keto diet, then you should try this lunch idea for sure!

Preparation time: 10 minutes
Cooking time: 30 minutes
Servings: 4

Ingredients:

- 1 yellow onion, chopped
- 1 pound carrots, sliced
- 1 tablespoon coconut oil
- Salt and black pepper to the taste
- 2 tablespoons ginger, minced
- 1 cup water
- 1 pound halibut, cut into medium chunks
- 12 cups chicken stock

Directions:

1. Heat up a pot with the oil over medium heat, add onion, stir and cook for 6 minutes.
2. Add ginger, carrots, water and stock, stir bring to a simmer, reduce temperature and cook for 20 minutes.

3. Blend soup using an immersion blender, season with salt and pepper and add halibut pieces.
4. Stir gently and simmer soup for 5 minutes more.
5. Divide into bowls and serve.

Enjoy!

Nutrition: calories 140, fat 6, fiber 1, carbs 4, protein 14

Simple Kimchi

Serve this with a steak!

Preparation time: 1 hour and 10 minutes
Cooking time: 0 minutes
Servings: 6

Ingredients:

- 3 tablespoons salt
- 1 pound napa cabbage, chopped
- 1 carrot, julienned
- ½ cup daikon radish
- 3 green onion stalks, chopped
- 1 tablespoon fish sauce
- 3 tablespoons chili flakes
- 3 garlic cloves, minced
- 1 tablespoon sesame oil
- ½ inch ginger, grated

Directions:

1. In a bowl, mix cabbage with the salt, massage well for 10 minutes, cover and leave aside for 1 hour.
2. In a bowl, mix chili flakes with fish sauce, garlic, sesame oil and ginger and stir very well.

3. Drain cabbage well, rinses under cold water and transfer to a bowl.
4. Add carrots, green onions, radish and chili paste and stir everything.
5. Leave in a dark and cold place for at least 2 days before serving as a side for a keto steak.

Enjoy!

Nutrition: calories 60, fat 3, fiber 2, carbs 5, protein 1

Delicious Green Beans Side Dish

You will definitely enjoy this great side dish!

Preparation time: 10 minutes

Cooking time: 10 minutes

Servings: 4

Ingredients:

- 2/3 cup parmesan, grated
- 1 egg
- 12 ounces green beans
- Salt and black pepper to the taste
- ½ teaspoon garlic powder
- ¼ teaspoon paprika

Directions:

1. In a bowl, mix parmesan with salt, pepper, garlic powder and paprika and stir.
2. In another bowl, whisk the egg with salt and pepper.
3. Dredge green beans in egg and then in parmesan mix.
4. Place green beans on a lined baking sheet, introduce in the oven at 400 degrees F for 10 minutes.
5. Serve hot as a side dish.

Enjoy!

Nutrition: calories 114, fat 5, fiber 7, carbs 3, protein 9

Simple Cauliflower Mash

This simple Ketogenic mash goes with a meat based dish!

Preparation time: 10 minutes
Cooking time: 10 minutes
Servings: 2

Ingredients:

- ¼ cup sour cream
- 1 small cauliflower head, florets separated
- Salt and black pepper to the taste
- 2 tablespoons feta cheese, crumbled
- 2 tablespoons black olives, pitted and sliced

Directions:

1. Put water in a pot, add some salt, bring to a boil over medium heat, add florets, cook for 10 minutes, take off heat and drain.
2. Return cauliflower to the pot, add salt and black pepper to the taste and the sour cream and blend suing an immersion blender.
3. Add black olives and feta cheese, stir and serve as a side dish.

Enjoy!

Nutrition: calories 100, fat 4, fiber 2, carbs 3, protein 2

Delicious Portobello Mushrooms

These are simply the best! It's a great keto side dish!

Preparation time: 10 minutes
Cooking time: 10 minutes
Servings: 4

Ingredients:

- 12 ounces Portobello mushrooms, sliced
- Salt and black pepper to the taste
- ½ teaspoon basil, dried
- 2 tablespoons olive oil
- ½ teaspoon tarragon, dried
- ½ teaspoon rosemary, dried
- ½ teaspoon thyme, dried
- 2 tablespoons balsamic vinegar

Directions:

1. In a bowl, mix oil with vinegar, salt, pepper, rosemary, tarragon, basil and thyme and whisk well.
2. Add mushroom slices, toss to coat well, place them on your preheated grill over medium high heat, cook for 5 minutes on both sides and serve as a keto side dish.

Enjoy!

Nutrition: calories 80, fat 4, fiber 4, carbs 2, protein 4

Brussels Sprouts Side Dish

This is an Asian-style side dish you must try!

Preparation time: 10 minutes
Cooking time: 10 minutes
Servings: 4

Ingredients:

- 1 pound Brussels sprouts, trimmed and halved
- Salt and black pepper to the taste
- 1 teaspoon sesame seeds
- 1 tablespoon green onions, chopped
- 1 and ½ tablespoons sukrin gold syrup
- 1 tablespoon coconut aminos
- 2 tablespoons sesame oil
- 1 tablespoon sriracha

Directions:

1. In a bowl, mix sesame oil with coconut aminos, sriracha, syrup, salt and black pepper and whisk well.
2. Heat up a pan over medium high heat, add Brussels sprouts and cook them for 5 minutes on each side.

3. Add sesame oil mix, toss to coat, sprinkle sesame seeds and green onions, stir again and serve as a side dish.

Enjoy!

Nutrition: calories 110, fat 4, fiber 4, carbs 6, protein 4

Delicious Pesto

This keto pesto can be served with a tasty chicken dish!

Preparation time: 10 minutes
Cooking time: 0 minutes
Servings: 4

Ingredients:

- ½ cup olive oil
- 2 cups basil
- 1/3 cup pine nuts
- 1/3 cup parmesan cheese, grated
- 2 garlic cloves, chopped
- Salt and black pepper to the taste

Directions:

1. Put basil in your food processor, add pine nuts and garlic and blend very well.
2. Add parmesan, salt, pepper and the oil gradually and blend again until you obtain a paste.
3. Serve with chicken!

Enjoy!

Nutrition: calories 100, fat 7, fiber 3, carbs 1, protein 5

Brussels Sprouts And Bacon

You will love Brussels sprouts from now on!

Preparation time: 10 minutes
Cooking time: 30 minutes
Servings: 4

Ingredients:

- 8 bacon strips, chopped
- 1 pound Brussels sprouts, trimmed and halved
- Salt and black pepper to the taste
- A pinch of cumin, ground
- A pinch of red pepper, crushed
- 2 tablespoons extra virgin olive oil

Directions:

1. In a bowl, mix Brussels sprouts with salt, pepper, cumin, red pepper and oil and toss to coat.
2. Spread Brussels sprouts on a lined baking sheet, introduce in the oven at 375 degrees F and bake for 30 minutes.
3. Meanwhile, heat up a pan over medium heat, add bacon pieces and cook them until they become crispy.

4. Divide baked Brussels sprouts on plates, top with bacon and serve as a side dish right away.

Enjoy!

Nutrition: calories 256, fat 20, fiber 6, carbs 5, protein 15

Delicious Spinach Side Dish

This is very creamy and tasty!

Preparation time: 10 minutes
Cooking time: 15 minutes
Servings: 2

Ingredients:

- 2 garlic cloves, minced
- 8 ounces spinach leaves
- A drizzle of olive oil
- Salt and black pepper to the taste
- 4 tablespoons sour cream
- 1 tablespoon ghee
- 2 tablespoons parmesan cheese, grated

Directions:

1. Heat up a pan with the oil over medium heat, add spinach, stir and cook until it softens.
2. Add salt, pepper, ghee, parmesan and ghee, stir and cook for 4 minutes.
3. Add sour cream, stir and cook for 5 minutes more.
4. Divide between plates and serve as a side dish.

Enjoy!

Nutrition: calories 133, fat 10, fiber 4, carbs 4, protein 2

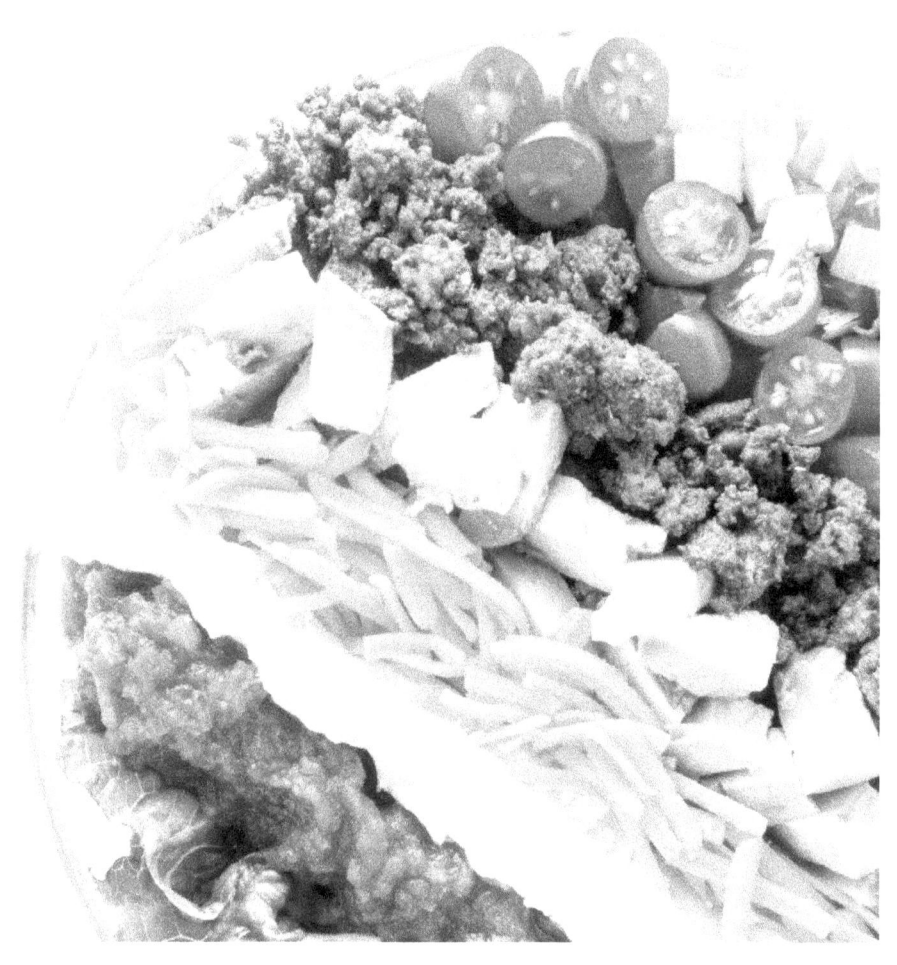

Amazing Avocado Fries

Try them as a side dish for a delicious steak!

Preparation time: 10 minutes
Cooking time: 5 minutes
Servings: 3

Ingredients:

- 3 avocados, pitted, peeled, halved and sliced
- 1 and ½ cups sunflower oil
- 1 and ½ cups almond meal
- A pinch of cayenne pepper
- Salt and black pepper to the taste

Directions:

1. In a bowl mix almond meal with salt, pepper and cayenne and stir.
2. In a second bowl, whisk eggs with a pinch of salt and pepper.
3. Dredge avocado pieces in egg and then in almond meal mix.
4. Heat up a pan with the oil over medium high heat, add avocado fries and cook them until they are golden.

5. Transfer to paper towels, drain grease and divide between plates.
6. Serve as a side dish.

Enjoy!

Nutrition: calories 450, fat 43, fiber 4, carbs 7, protein 17

Simple Roasted Cauliflower

This is so delicious and very easy to make at home! It's a great keto side dish!

Preparation time: 10 minutes
Cooking time: 25 minutes
Servings: 6

Ingredients:

- 1 cauliflower head, florets separated
- Salt and black pepper to the taste
- 1/3 cup parmesan, grated
- 1 tablespoon parsley, chopped
- 3 tablespoons olive oil
- 2 tablespoons extra virgin olive oil

Directions:

1. In a bowl, mix oil with garlic, salt, pepper and cauliflower florets.
2. Toss to coat well, spread this on a lined baking sheet, introduce in the oven at 450 degrees F and bake for 25 minutes, stirring halfway.

3. Add parmesan and parsley, stir and cook for 5 minutes more.
4. Divide between plates and serve as a keto side dish. Enjoy!

Nutrition: calories 118, fat 2, fiber 3, carbs 1, protein 6

Mushroom And Spinach Side Dish

This is an Italian style keto side dish worth trying as soon as possible!

Preparation time: 10 minutes
Cooking time: 10 minutes
Servings: 4

Ingredients:

- 10 ounces spinach leaves, chopped
- Salt and black pepper to the taste
- 14 ounces mushrooms, chopped
- 2 garlic cloves, minced
- A handful parsley, chopped
- 1 yellow onion, chopped
- 4 tablespoons olive oil
- 2 tablespoons balsamic vinegar

Directions:

1. Heat up a pan with the oil over medium high heat, add garlic and onion, stir and cook for 4 minutes.
2. Add mushrooms, stir and cook for 3 minutes more.
3. Add spinach, stir and cook for 3 minutes.

4. Add vinegar, salt and pepper, stir and cook for 1 minute more.
5. Add parsley, stir, divide between plates and serve hot as a side dish.

Enjoy!

Nutrition: calories 200, fat 4, fiber 6, carbs 2, protein 12

Delicious Okra And Tomatoes

This is very simple and easy to make! It's one of the best keto sides ever!

Preparation time: 10 minutes
Cooking time: 10 minutes
Servings: 6

Ingredients:

- 14 ounces canned stewed tomatoes, chopped
- Salt and black pepper to the taste
- 2 celery stalks, chopped
- 1 yellow onion, chopped
- 1 pound okra, sliced
- 2 bacon slices, chopped
- 1 small green bell peppers, chopped

Directions:

1. Heat up a pan over medium high heat, add bacon, stir, brown for a few minutes, transfer to paper towels and leave aside for now.
2. Heat up the pan again over medium heat, add okra, bell pepper, onion and celery, stir and cook for 2 minutes.

3. Add tomatoes, salt and pepper, stir and cook for 3 minutes.
4. Divide on plates, garnish with crispy bacon and serve. Enjoy!

Nutrition: calories 100, fat 2, fiber 3, carbs 2, protein 6

Amazing Snap Peas And Mint

This side dish is not just a keto one! It's a simple and quick one as well!

Preparation time: 10 minutes
Cooking time: 5 minutes
Servings: 4

Ingredients:

- ¾ pound sugar snap peas, trimmed
- Salt and black pepper to the taste
- 1 tablespoon mint leaves, chopped
- 2 teaspoons olive oil
- 3 green onions, chopped
- 1 garlic clove, minced

Directions:

1. Heat up a pan with the oil over medium high heat.
2. Add snap peas, salt, pepper, green onions, garlic and mint.
3. Stir everything, cook for 5 minutes, divide between plates and serve as a side dish for a pork steak.

Enjoy!

Nutrition: calories 70, fat 1, fiber 1, carbs 0.4, protein 6

Collard Greens Side Dish

This is just unbelievably amazing!

Preparation time: 10 minutes
Cooking time: 2 hours and 15 minutes
Servings: 10

Ingredients:

- 5 bunches collard greens, chopped
- Salt and black pepper to the taste
- 1 tablespoon red pepper flakes, crushed
- 5 cups chicken stock
- 1 turkey leg
- 2 tablespoons garlic, minced
- ¼ cup olive oil

Directions:

1. Heat up a pot with the oil over medium heat, add garlic, stir and cook for 1 minute.
2. Add stock, salt, pepper and turkey leg, stir, cover and simmer for 30 minutes.
3. Add collard greens, cover pot again and cook for 45 minutes more.

4. Reduce heat to medium, add more salt and pepper, stir and cook for 1 hour.
5. Drain greens, mix them with red pepper flakes, stir, divide between plates and serve as a side dish.

Enjoy!

Nutrition: calories 143, fat 3, fiber 4, carbs 3, protein 6

Eggplant And Tomato Side Dish

It's a keto side dish you will make over and over again!

Preparation time: 10 minutes
Cooking time: 15 minutes
Servings: 4

Ingredients:

- 1 tomato, sliced
- 1 eggplant, sliced into thin rounds
- Salt and black pepper to the taste
- ¼ cup parmesan, grated
- A drizzle of olive oil

Directions:

1. Place eggplant slices on a lined baking dish, drizzle some oil and sprinkle half of the parmesan.
2. Top eggplant slices with tomato ones, season with salt and pepper to the taste and sprinkle the rest of the cheese over them.
3. Introduce in the oven at 400 degrees F and bake for 15 minutes.
4. Divide between plates and serve hot as a side dish.

Enjoy!

Nutrition: calories 55, fat 1, fiber 1, carbs 0.5, protein 7

Broccoli With Lemon Almond Butter

This side dish is perfect for a grilled steak!

Preparation time: 10 minutes
Cooking time: 10 minutes
Servings: 4

Ingredients:

- 1 broccoli head, florets separated
- Salt and black pepper to the taste
- ¼ cup almonds, blanched
- 1 teaspoon lemon zest
- ¼ cup coconut butter, melted
- 2 tablespoons lemon juice

Directions:

1. Put water in a pot, add salt and bring to a boil over medium high heat.
2. Place broccoli florets in a steamer basket, place into the pot, cover and steam for 8 minutes.
3. Drain and transfer to a bowl.

4. Heat up a pan with the coconut butter over medium heat, add lemon juice, lemon zest and almonds, stir and take off heat.
5. Add broccoli, toss to coat, divide between plates and serve as a Ketogenic side dish.

Enjoy!

Nutrition: calories 170, fat 15, fiber 4, carbs 4, protein 4

Delicious Pesto Crackers

It's one of the tastiest keto snacks ever!

Preparation time: 10 minutes
Cooking time: 17 minutes
Servings: 6

Ingredients:

- ½ teaspoon baking powder
- Salt and black pepper to the taste
- 1 and ¼ cups almond flour
- ¼ teaspoon basil, dried
- 1 garlic clove, minced
- 2 tablespoons basil pesto
- A pinch of cayenne pepper
- 3 tablespoons ghee

Directions:

1. In a bowl, mix salt, pepper, baking powder and almond flour.
2. Add garlic, cayenne and basil and stir.
3. Add pesto and whisk.
4. Also add ghee and mix your dough with your finger.

5. Spread this dough on a lined baking sheet, introduce in the oven at 325 degrees F and bake for 17 minutes.
6. Leave aside to cool down, cut your crackers and serve them as a snack.

Enjoy!

Nutrition: calories 200, fat 20, fiber 1, carbs 4, protein 7

Pumpkin Muffins

You can even take this snack at the office!

Preparation time: 10 minutes
Cooking time: 15 minutes
Servings: 18

Ingredients:

- ¼ cup sunflower seed butter
- ¾ cup pumpkin puree
- 2 tablespoons flaxseed meal
- ¼ cup coconut flour
- ½ cup erythritol
- ½ teaspoon nutmeg, ground
- 1 teaspoon cinnamon, ground
- ½ teaspoon baking soda
- 1 egg
- ½ teaspoon baking powder
- A pinch of salt

Directions:

1. In a bowl, mix butter with pumpkin puree and egg and blend well.
2. Add flaxseed meal, coconut flour, erythritol, baking soda, baking powder, nutmeg, cinnamon and a pinch of salt and stir well.
3. Spoon this into a greased muffin pan, introduce in the oven at 350 degrees F and bake for 15 minutes.
4. Leave muffins to cool down and serve them as a snack. Enjoy!

Nutrition: calories 50, fat 3, fiber 1, carbs 2, protein 2

Delicious Bombs

This snack is easy to make! Try it!

Preparation time: 10 minutes
Cooking time: 0 minutes
Servings: 6

Ingredients:

- 8 black olives, pitted and chopped
- Salt and black pepper to the taste
- 2 tablespoons sun-dried tomato pesto
- 14 pepperoni slices, chopped
- 4 ounces cream cheese
- 1 tablespoons basil, chopped

Directions:
1. In a bowl, mix cream cheese with salt, pepper, pepperoni, basil, sun dried tomato pesto and black olives and stir well.
2. Shape balls from this mix, arrange on a platter and serve.

Enjoy!

Nutrition: calories 110, fat 10, fiber 0, carbs 1.4, protein 3

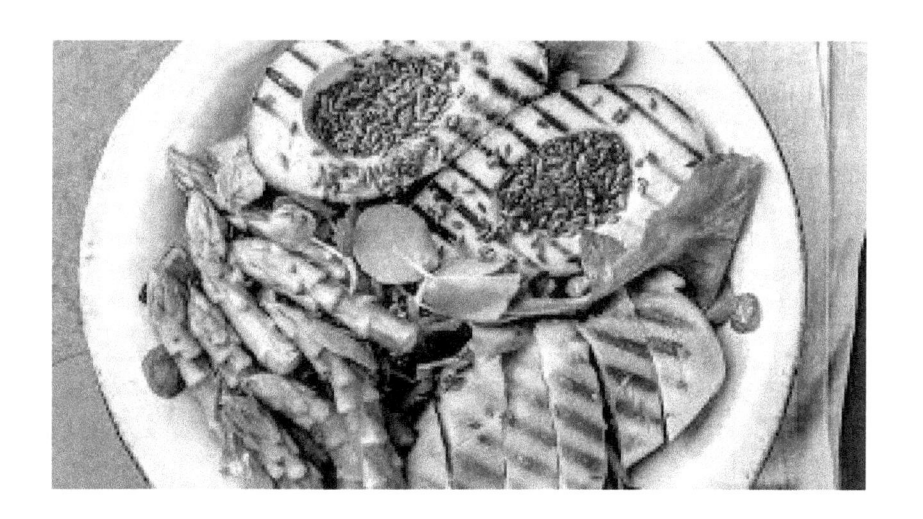

Special Tortilla Chips

It's an exceptional keto snack recipe!

Preparation time: 10 minutes
Cooking time: 14 minutes
Servings: 6

Ingredients:

For the tortillas:

- 2 teaspoons olive oil
- 1 cup flax seed meal
- 2 tablespoons psyllium husk powder
- ¼ teaspoon xanthan gum
- 1 cup water
- ½ teaspoon curry powder
- 3 teaspoons coconut flour

For the chips:

- 6 flaxseed tortillas
- Salt and black pepper to the taste
- 3 tablespoons vegetable oil
- Fresh salsa for serving
- Sour cream for serving

Directions:

1. In a bowl, mix flaxseed meal with psyllium powder, olive oil, xanthan gum, water and curry powder and mix until you obtain an elastic dough.
2. Spread coconut flour on a working surface.
3. Divide dough into 6 pieces, place each piece on the working surface and roll into a circle and cut each into 6 pieces.
4. Heat up a pan with the vegetable oil over medium high heat, add tortilla chips, cook for 2 minutes on each side and transfer to paper towels.
5. Put tortilla chips in a bowl, season with salt and pepper and serve with some fresh salsa and sour cream on the side.

Enjoy!

Nutrition: calories 30, fat 3, fiber 1.2, carbs 0.5, protein 1

Amazing Jalapeno Balls

These are easy to make but they are so flavored and delicious!

Preparation time: 10 minutes

Cooking time: 10 minutes

Servings: 3

Ingredients:

- 3 bacon slices
- 3 ounces cream cheese
- ¼ teaspoon onion powder
- Salt and black pepper to the taste
- 1 jalapeno pepper, chopped
- ½ teaspoon parsley, dried
- ¼ teaspoon garlic powder

Directions:
1. Heat up a pan over medium high heat, add bacon, cook until it's crispy, transfer to paper towels, drain grease and crumble.
2. Reserve bacon fat from the pan.
3. In a bowl, mix cream cheese with jalapeno pepper, onion and garlic powder, parsley, salt and pepper and stir well.
4. Add bacon fat and bacon crumbles, stir gently, shape balls from this mix and serve.

Enjoy!

Nutrition: calories 200, fat 18, fiber 1, carbs 2, protein 5

Cheeseburger Muffins

This is a great keto appetizer for a sports night!

Preparation time: 10 minutes
Cooking time: 30 minutes
Servings: 9

Ingredients:

- ½ cup flaxseed meal
- ½ cup almond flour
- Salt and black pepper to the taste
- 2 eggs
- 1 teaspoon baking powder
- ¼ cups sour cream

For the filling:

- ½ teaspoon onion powder
- 16 ounces beef, ground
- Salt and black pepper to the taste
- 2 tablespoons tomato paste
- ½ teaspoon garlic powder
- ½ cup cheddar cheese, grated
- 2 tablespoons mustard

Directions:
1. In a bowl, mix almond flour with flaxseed meal, salt, pepper and baking powder and whisk.
2. Add eggs and sour cream and stir very well.
3. Divide this into a greased muffin pan and press well using your fingers.
4. Heat up a pan over medium high heat, add beef, stir and brown for a few minutes.
5. Add salt, pepper, onion powder, garlic powder and tomato paste and stir well.
6. Cook for 5 minutes more and take off heat.
7. Fill cupcakes crusts with this mix, introduce in the oven at 350 degrees F and bake for 15 minutes.
8. Spread cheese on top, introduce in the oven again and bake muffins for 5 minutes more.
9. Serve with mustard and your favorite toppings on top.

Enjoy!

Nutrition: calories 245, fat 16, fiber 6, carbs 2, protein 14

Tasty Pizza Dip

You will love this great dip!

Preparation time: 10 minutes
Cooking time: 20 minutes
Servings: 4

Ingredients:

- 4 ounces cream cheese, soft
- ½ cup mozzarella cheese
- ¼ cup sour cream
- Salt and black pepper to the taste
- 1/2 cup tomato sauce
- ¼ cup mayonnaise
- ¼ cup parmesan cheese, grated
- 1 tablespoon green bell pepper, chopped
- 6 pepperoni slices, chopped
- ½ teaspoon Italian seasoning
- 4 black olives, pitted and chopped

Directions:

1. In a bowl, mix cream cheese with mozzarella, sour cream, mayo, salt and pepper and stir well.
2. Spread this into 4 ramekins, add a layer of tomato sauce, then layer parmesan cheese, top with bell pepper, pepperoni, Italian seasoning and black olives.
3. Introduce in the oven at 350 degrees F and bake for 20 minutes.
4. Serve warm.

Enjoy!

Nutrition: calories 400, fat 34, fiber 4, carbs 4, protein 15

Incredible Keto Muffins Snack

Everyone appreciates a great treat! Try this one soon!

Preparation time: 10 minutes

Cooking time: 15 minutes

Servings: 20

Ingredients:

- ½ cup flaxseed meal
- ½ cup almond flour
- 3 tablespoons swerve
- 1 tablespoon psyllium powder
- A pinch of salt
- Cooking spray
- ¼ teaspoon baking powder
- 1 egg
- ¼ cup coconut milk
- 1/3 cup sour cream
- 3 hot dogs, cut into 20 pieces

Directions:
1. In a bowl, mix flaxseed meal with flour, psyllium powder, swerve, salt and baking powder and stir.
2. Add egg, sour cream and coconut milk and whisk well.
3. Grease a muffin tray with cooking oil, divide the batter you've just make, stick a hot dog piece in the middle of each muffin, introduce in the oven at 350 degrees F and bake for 12 minutes.
4. Broil in preheated broil for 3 minutes more, divide on a platter and serve.

Enjoy!

Nutrition: calories 80, fat 6, fiber 1, carbs 1, protein 3

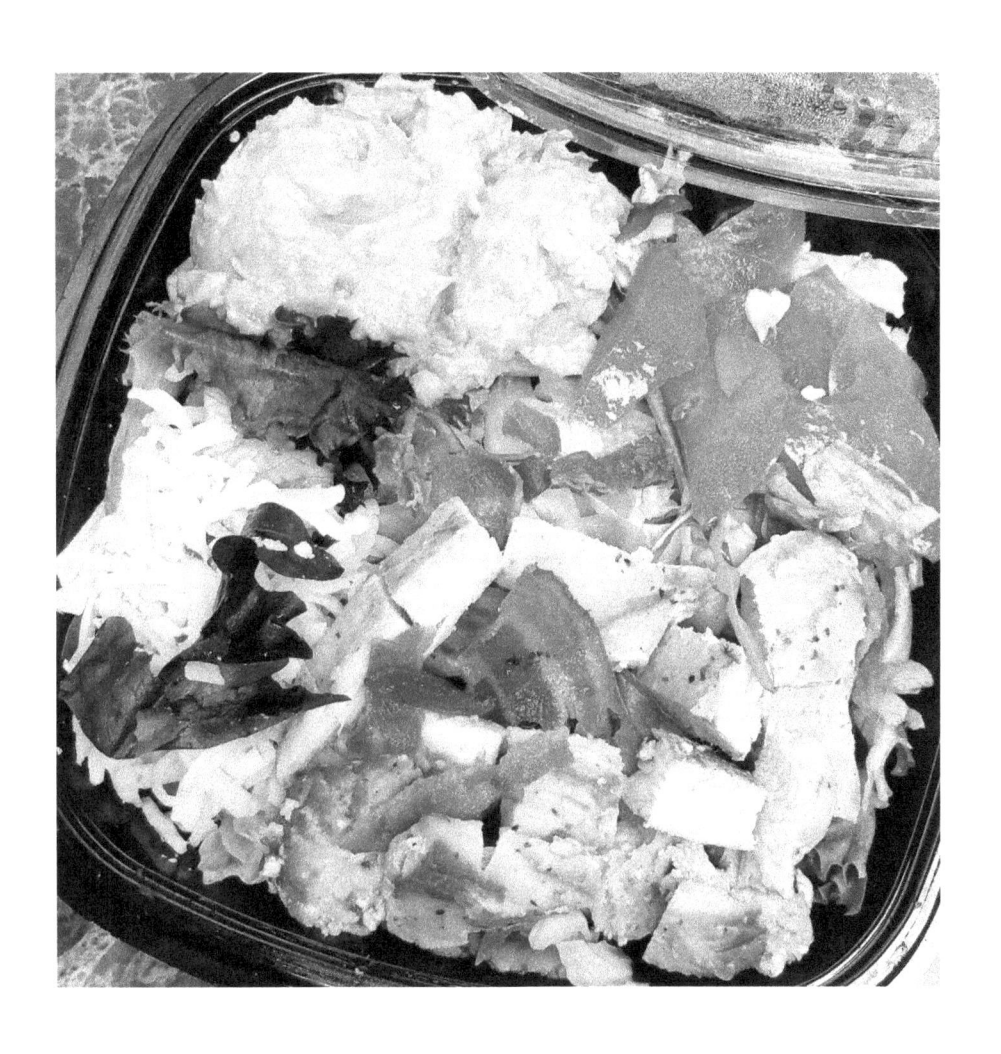

Amazing Fried Queso Snack

It's a crispy and tasty keto snack!

Preparation time: 10 minutes
Cooking time: 10 minutes
Servings: 6

Ingredients:

- 2 ounces olives, pitted and chopped
- 5 ounces queso Blanco, cubed and freeze for a couple of minutes
- A pinch of red pepper flakes
- 1 and ½ tablespoons olive oil

Directions:

1. Heat up a pan with the oil over medium high heat, add queso cubes and cook until the bottom melts a bit.
2. Flip cubes with a spatula and sprinkle black olives on top.
3. Leave cubes to cook a bit more, flip and sprinkle red pepper flakes and cook until they are crispy.

4. Flip, cook on the other side until it's crispy as well, transfer to a cutting board, cut into small blocks and then serve as a snack.

Enjoy!

Nutrition: calories 500, fat 43, fiber 4, carbs 2, protein 30

Maple And Pecan Bars

This is a very healthy keto snack for you to try soon!

Preparation time: 10 minutes
Cooking time: 25 minutes
Servings: 12

Ingredients:

- ½ cup flaxseed meal
- 2 cups pecans, toasted and crushed
- 1 cup almond flour
- ½ cup coconut oil
- ¼ teaspoon stevia
- ½ cup coconut, shredded
- ¼ cup "maple syrup"

For the maple syrup:

- ¼ cup erythritol
- 2 and ¼ teaspoons coconut oil
- 1 tablespoon ghee
- ¼ teaspoon xanthan gum
- ¾ cup water
- 2 teaspoons maple extract

- ½ teaspoon vanilla extract

Directions:
1. In a heatproof bowl, mix ghee with 2 and ¼ teaspoons coconut oil and xanthan gum, stir, introduce in your microwave and heat up for 1 minute.
2. Add erythritol, water, maple and vanilla extract, stir well and heat up in the microwave for 1 minute more.
3. In a bowl, mix flaxseed meal with coconut and almond flour and stir.
4. Add pecans and stir again.
5. Add ¼ cup "maple syrup", stevia and ½ cup coconut oil and stir well.
6. Spread this in a baking dish, press well, introduce in the oven at 350 degrees F and bake for 25 minutes.
7. Leave aside to cool down, cut into 12 bars and serve as a keto snack.

Enjoy!

Nutrition: calories 300, fat 30, fiber 12, carbs 2, protein 5

Summer Side Salad

It's going to be the best summer side salad ever!

Preparation time: 10 minutes

Cooking time: 5 minutes

Servings: 6

Ingredients:

- ½ cup extra virgin olive oil
- 1 cucumber, chopped
- 2 baguettes, cut into small cubes
- 2 pints colored cherry tomatoes, cut in halves
- Salt and black pepper to the taste
- 1 red onion, chopped
- 3 tablespoons balsamic vinegar
- 1 garlic clove, minced
- 1 bunch basil, roughly chopped

Directions:

1. In a bowl, mix bread cubes with half of the oil and toss to coat.

2. Heat up a pan over medium high heat, add bread, stir, toast for 10 minutes, take off heat, drain and leave aside for now.
3. In a bowl, mix vinegar with salt, pepper and the rest of the oil and whisk very well.
4. In a salad bowl mix cucumber with tomatoes, onion, garlic and bread.
5. Add vinegar dressing, toss to coat, sprinkle basil, add more salt and pepper if needed, toss to coat and serve.

Enjoy!

Nutrition: calories 90, fat 0, fiber 2, carbs 2, protein 4

Tomato And Bocconcini

This salad goes really well with a grilled steak!

Preparation time: 6 minutes
Cooking time: 0 minutes
Servings: 4

Ingredients:

- 20 ounces tomatoes, cut in wedges
- 2 tablespoons extra virgin olive oil
- 1 and ½ tablespoons balsamic vinegar
- 1 teaspoon stevia
- 1 garlic clove, finely minced
- 8 ounces baby bocconcini, drain and torn
- 1 cup basil leaves, roughly chopped
- Salt and black pepper to the taste

Directions:

1. In a bowl, mix stevia with vinegar, garlic, oil, salt and pepper and whisk very well.
2. In a salad bowl, mix bocconcini with tomato and basil.
3. Add dressing, toss to coat and serve right away as a keto side dish.

Enjoy!

Nutrition: calories 100, fat 2, fiber 2, carbs 1, protein 9

Cucumber And Dates Salad

This is a very healthy keto side salad! Try it and enjoy its taste!

Preparation time: 10 minutes

Cooking time: 0 minutes

Servings: 4

Ingredients:

- 2 English cucumbers, chopped
- 8 dates, pitted and sliced
- ¾ cup fennel, thinly sliced
- 2 tablespoons chives, finely chopped
- ½ cup walnuts, chopped
- 2 tablespoons lemon juice
- 4 tablespoons fruity olive oil
- Salt and black pepper to the taste

Directions:

1. Put cucumber pieces on a paper towel, press well and transfer to a salad bowl.
2. Crush them a bit using a fork.
3. Add dates, fennel, chives and walnuts and stir gently.

4. Add salt, pepper to the taste, lemon juice and the oil, toss to coat and serve right away.

Enjoy!

Nutrition: calories 80, fat 0.2, fiber 1, carbs 0.4, protein 5

Easy Eggplant Salad

It's a good idea for a light keto side dish!

Preparation time: 10 minutes

Cooking time: 10 minutes

Servings: 4

Ingredients:

- 1 eggplant, sliced
- 1 red onion, sliced
- A drizzle of canola oil
- 1 avocado, pitted and chopped
- 1 teaspoon mustard
- 1 tablespoon balsamic vinegar
- 1 tablespoon fresh oregano, chopped
- A drizzle of olive oil
- Salt and black pepper to the taste
- Zest from 1 lemon
- Some parsley sprigs, chopped for serving

Directions:

1. Brush red onion slices and eggplant ones with a drizzle of canola oil, place them on heated kitchen grill and cook them until they become soft.
2. Transfer them to a cutting board, leave them to cool down, chop them and put them in a bowl.
3. Add avocado and stir gently.
4. In a bowl, mix vinegar with mustard, oregano, olive oil, salt and pepper to the taste.
5. Add this to eggplant, avocado and onion mix, toss to coat, add lemon zest and parsley on top and serve.

Enjoy!

Nutrition: calories 120, fat 3, fiber 2, carbs 1, protein 8

Special Side Salad

We really like this Italian style side salad!

Preparation time: 2 hours and 10 minutes
Cooking time: 1 hour and 30 minutes
Servings: 12

Ingredients:

- 1 garlic clove, crushed
- 6 eggplants
- 1 teaspoon parsley, dried
- 1 teaspoon oregano, dried
- ¼ teaspoon basil, dried
- 3 tablespoons extra virgin olive oil
- 2 tablespoons stevia
- 1 tablespoon balsamic vinegar
- Salt and black pepper to the taste

Directions:

1. Prick eggplants with a fork, arrange them on a baking sheet, introduce in the oven at 350 degrees F, bake for 1 hour and 30 minutes, take them out of the oven, leave

them to cool down, peel, chop them and transfer to a salad bowl.
2. Add garlic, oil, parsley, stevia, oregano, basil, salt and pepper to the taste, toss to coat, keep in the fridge for 2 hours and then serve.

Enjoy!

Nutrition: calories 150, fat 1, fiber 2, carbs 1, protein 8

Special Endives And Watercress Side Salad

It's such a fresh side dish that goes with a keto grilled steak!

Preparation time: 10 minutes

Cooking time: 5 minutes

Servings: 4

Ingredients:

- 4 medium endives, roots and ends cut and thinly sliced crosswise
- 1 tablespoon lemon juice
- 1 shallot finely, chopped
- 1 tablespoon balsamic vinegar
- 2 tablespoons extra virgin olive oil
- 6 tablespoons heavy cream
- Salt and black pepper to the taste
- 4 ounces watercress, cut in medium springs
- 1 apple, thinly sliced
- 1 tablespoon chervil, chopped
- 1 tablespoon tarragon, chopped
- 1 tablespoon chives, chopped
- 1/3 cup almonds, chopped
- 1 tablespoon parsley, chopped

Directions:
1. In a bowl, mix lemon juice with vinegar, salt and shallot, stir and leave a side for 10 minutes.
2. Add olive oil, pepper, stir and leave aside for another 2 minutes.
3. Put endives, apple, watercress, chives, tarragon, parsley and chervil in a salad bowl.
4. Add salt and pepper to the taste and toss to coat.
5. Add heavy cream and vinaigrette, stir gently and serve as a side dish with almonds on top.

Enjoy!

Nutrition: calories 200, fat 3, fiber 5, carbs 2, protein 10

Indian Side Salad

It's very healthy and rich!

Preparation time: 15 minutes
Cooking time: 0 minutes
Servings: 6

Ingredients:

- 3 carrots, finely grated
- 2 courgettes, finely sliced
- A bunch of radishes, finely sliced
- ½ red onion, chopped
- 6 mint leaves, roughly chopped

For the salad dressing:

- 1 teaspoon mustard
- 1 tablespoons homemade mayo
- 1 tablespoons balsamic vinegar
- 2 tablespoons extra virgin olive oil
- Salt and black pepper to the taste

Directions:

1. In a bowl, mix mustard with mayo, vinegar, salt and pepper to the taste and stir well.

2. Add oil gradually and whisk everything.
3. In a salad bowl, mix carrots with radishes, courgettes and mint leaves.
4. Add salad dressing, toss to coat and keep in the fridge until you serve it.

Enjoy!

Nutrition: calories 140, fat 1, fiber 2, carbs 1, protein 7

Indian Mint Chutney

It has such a unique color and taste! It's a special side for any steak!

Preparation time: 10 minutes
Cooking time: 0 minutes
Servings: 8

Ingredients:

- 1 and ½ cup mint leaves
- 1 big bunch cilantro
- Salt and black pepper to the taste
- 1 green chili pepper, seedless
- 1 yellow onion, cut into medium chunks
- ¼ cup water
- 1 tablespoon tamarind juice

Directions:

1. Put mint and coriander leaves in your food processor and blend them.
2. Add chili pepper, salt, black pepper, onion and tamarind paste and blend again.

3. Add water, blend some more until you obtain cream, transfer to a bowl and serve as a side for a tasty keto steak.

Enjoy!

Nutrition: calories 100, fat 1, fiber 1, carbs 0.4, protein 6

Indian Coconut Chutney

It's perfect for a fancy Indian style Ketogenic dish!

Preparation time: 5 minutes

Cooking time: 5 minutes

Servings: 3

Ingredients:

- ½ teaspoon cumin
- ½ cup coconut, grated
- 2 tablespoons already fried chana dal
- 2 green chilies
- Salt to the taste
- 1 garlic clove
- ¾ tablespoons avocado oil
- ¼ teaspoon mustard seeds
- A pinch of hing
- ½ teaspoons urad dal
- 1 red chili chopped
- 1 spring curry leaves

Directions:

1. In your food processor, mix coconut with salt to the taste, cumin, garlic, chana dal and green chilies and blend well.
2. Add a splash of water and blend again.
3. Heat up a pan with the oil over medium heat, add red chili, urad dal, mustard seeds, hing and curry leaves, stir and cook for 2-3 minutes.
4. Add this to coconut chutney, stir gently and serve as a side.

Enjoy!

Nutrition: calories 90, fat 1, fiber 1, carbs 1, protein 6

Easy Tamarind Chutney

It's sweet and it's perfectly balanced! It's one of the best sides for a keto dish!

Preparation time: 10 minutes
Cooking time: 35 minutes
Servings: 10

Ingredients:

- 1 teaspoon cumin seeds
- 1 tablespoon canola oil
- ½ teaspoon garam masala
- ½ teaspoon asafetida powder
- 1 teaspoon ground ginger
- ½ teaspoon fennel seeds
- ½ teaspoon cayenne pepper
- 1 and ¼ cups coconut sugar
- 2 cups water
- 3 tablespoons tamarind paste

Directions:

1. Heat up a pan with the oil over medium heat, add ginger, cumin, cayenne pepper, asafetida powder,

fennel seeds and garam masala, stir and cook for 2 minutes.
2. Add water, sugar and tamarind paste, stir, bring to a boil, reduce heat to low and simmer chutney for 30 minutes.
3. Transfer to a bowl and leave it to cool down before you serve it as a side for a steak.

Enjoy!

Nutrition: calories 120, fat 1, fiber 3, carbs 5, protein 9

Caramelized Bell Peppers

A Ketogenic pork dish will taste much better with such a side dish!

Preparation time: 10 minutes
Cooking time: 32 minutes
Servings: 4

Ingredients:

- 1 tablespoon olive oil
- 1 teaspoon ghee
- 2 red bell peppers, cut into thin strips
- 2 red onions, cut into thin strips
- Salt and black pepper to the taste
- 1 teaspoon basil, dried

Directions:

1. Heat up a pan with the ghee and the oil over medium heat, add onion and bell peppers, stir and cook for 2 minutes.
2. Reduce temperature and cook for 30 minutes more stirring often.
3. Add salt, pepper and basil, stir again, take off heat and serve as a keto side dish.

Enjoy!

Nutrition: calories 97, fat 4, fiber 2, carbs 6, protein 2

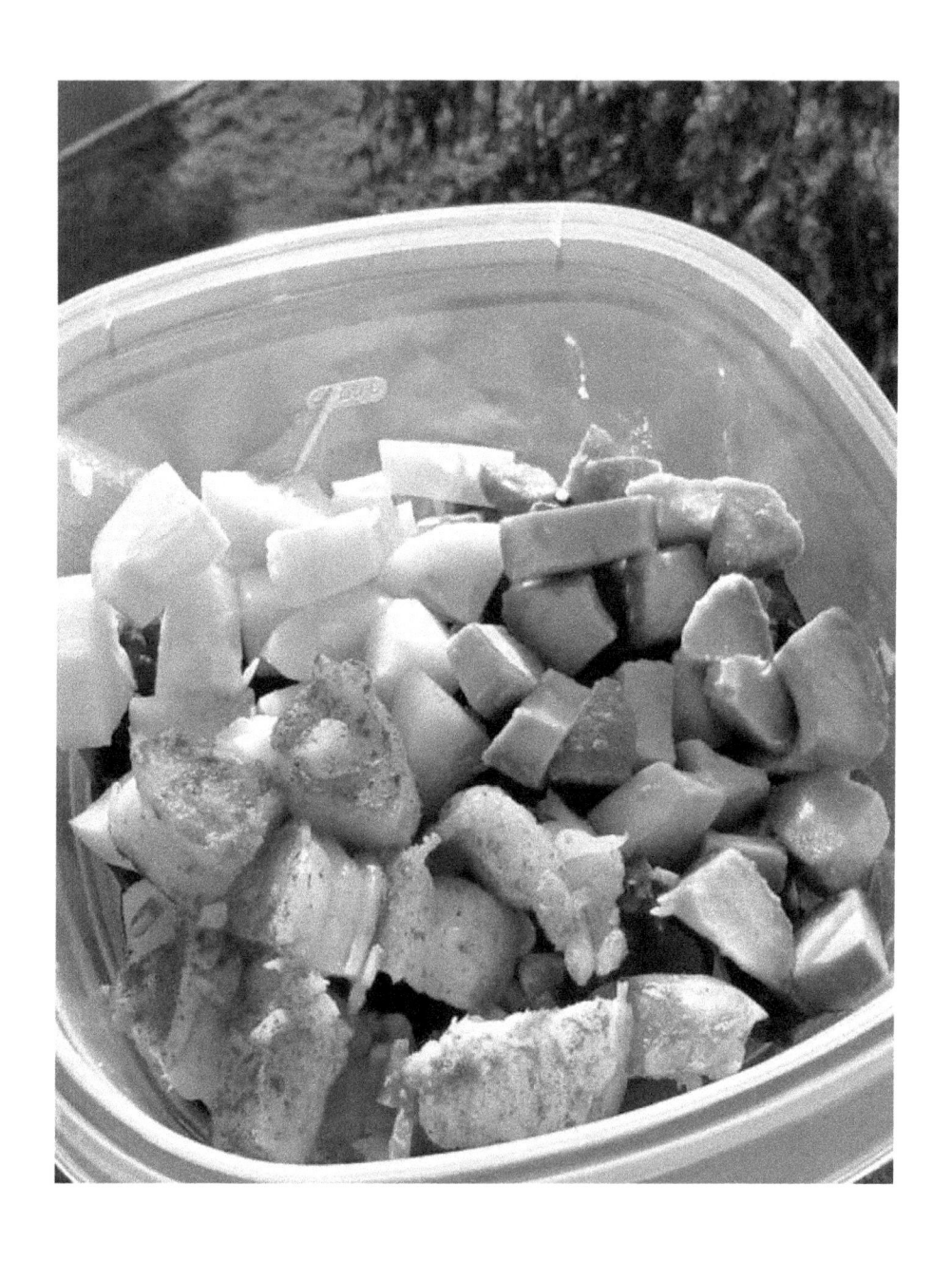

Caramelized Red Chard

This is an easy side for a dinner dish!

Preparation time: 10 minutes
Cooking time: 20 minutes
Servings: 4

Ingredients:

- 2 tablespoons olive oil
- 1 yellow onion, chopped
- 2 tablespoons capers
- Juice of 1 lemon
- Salt and black pepper to the taste
- 1 teaspoon palm sugar
- 1 bunch red chard, chopped
- ¼ cup kalamata olives, pitted and chopped

Directions:

1. Heat up a pan with the oil over medium heat, add onions, stir and brown for 4 minutes.
2. Add palm sugar and stir well.
3. Add olives and chard, stir and cook for 10 minutes more.

4. Add capers, lemon juice, salt and pepper, stir and cook for 3 minutes more.
5. Divide between plates and serve as a keto side. Enjoy!

Nutrition: calories 119, fat 7, fiber 3, carbs 7, protein 2

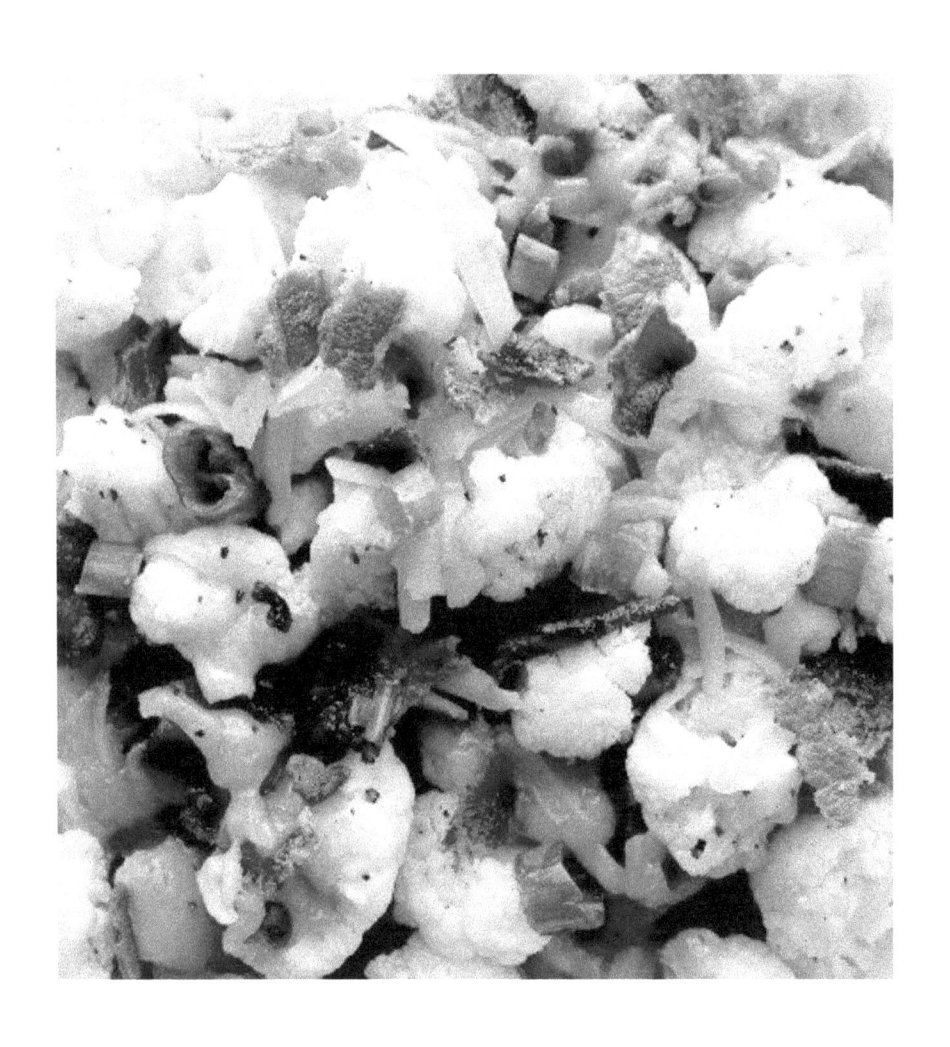

Conclusion

This is really a life changing cookbook. It shows you everything you need to know about the Ketogenic diet and it helps you get started.

You now know some of the best and most popular Ketogenic recipes in the world.

We have something for everyone's taste!

So, don't hesitate too much and start your new life as a follower of the Ketogenic diet!

Get your hands on this special recipes collection and start cooking in this new, exciting and healthy way!

Have a lot of fun and enjoy your Ketogenic diet!

Avocado Dip

This is not a guacamole but it's equally delicious!

Preparation time: 3 hours and 10 minutes
Cooking time: 10 minutes
Servings: 4

Ingredients:

- ¼ cup erythritol powder
- 2 avocados, pitted, peeled and cut into slices
- ¼ teaspoon stevia
- ½ cup cilantro, chopped
- Juice and zest of 2 limes
- 1 cup coconut milk

Directions:

1. Place avocado slices on a lined baking sheet, squeeze half of the lime juice over them and keep in your freezer for 3 hours.
2. Heat up the coconut milk in a pan over medium heat.
3. Add lime zest, stir and bring to a boil.
4. Add erythritol powder, stir, take off heat and leave aside to cool down a bit.

5. Transfer avocado to your food processor, add the rest of the lime juice and the cilantro and pulse well.
6. Add coconut milk mix and stevia and blend well.
7. Transfer to a bowl and serve right away.

Enjoy!

Nutrition: calories 150, fat 14, fiber 2, carbs 4, protein 2

Special Prosciutto And Shrimp Appetizer

You've got to love this! It's tasty!

Preparation time: 10 minutes
Cooking time: 20 minutes
Servings: 16

Ingredients:

- 2 tablespoons olive oil
- 10 ounces already cooked shrimp, peeled and deveined
- 1 tablespoons mint, chopped
- 2 tablespoons erythritol
- 1/3 cup blackberries, ground
- 11 prosciutto sliced
- 1/3 cup red wine

Directions:

1. Wrap each shrimp in prosciutto slices, arrange on a lined baking sheet, drizzle the olive oil over them, introduce in the oven at 425 degrees F and bake for 15 minutes.

2. Heat up a pan with ground blackberries over medium heat, add mint, wine and erythritol, stir, cook for 3 minutes and take off heat.
3. Arrange shrimp on a platter, drizzle blackberries sauce over them and serve.

Enjoy!

Nutrition: calories 245, fat 12, fiber 2, carbs 1, protein 14

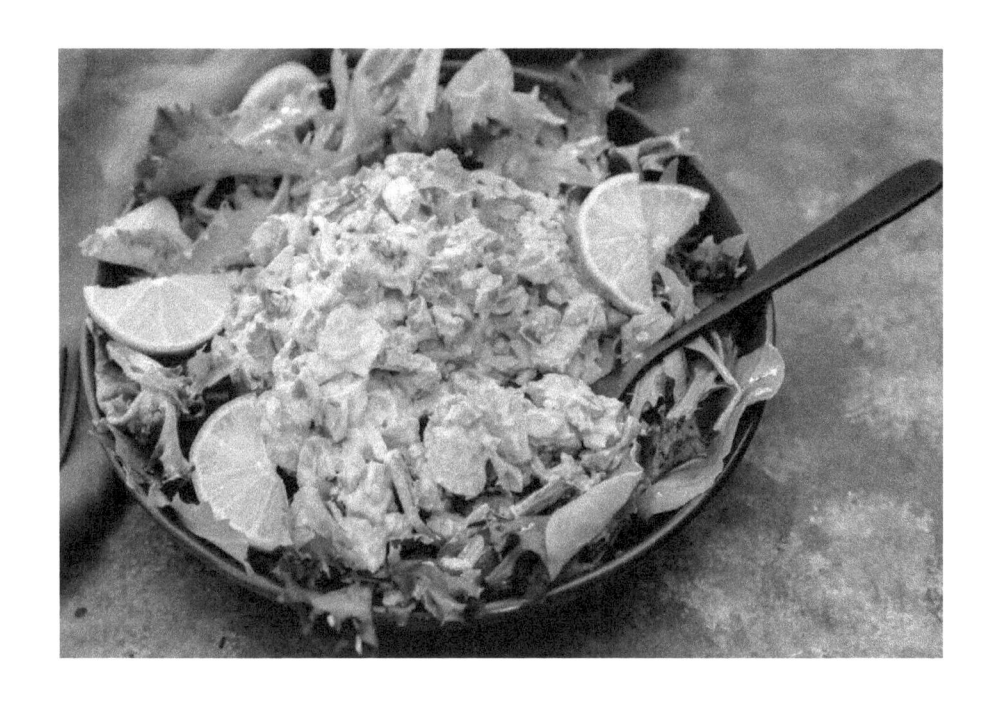

Broccoli And Cheddar Biscuits

This snack will really make you feel full for a couple of hours!

Preparation time: 10 minutes
Cooking time: 25 minutes
Servings: 12

Ingredients:

- 4 cups broccoli florets
- 1 and ½ cup almond flour
- 1 teaspoon paprika
- Salt and black pepper to the taste
- 2 eggs
- ¼ cup coconut oil
- 2 cups cheddar cheese, grated
- 1 teaspoon garlic powder
- ½ teaspoon apple cider vinegar
- ½ teaspoon baking soda

Directions:

1. Put broccoli florets in your food processor, add some salt and pepper and blend well.

2. In a bowl, mix almond flour with salt, pepper, paprika, garlic powder and baking soda and stir.
3. Add cheddar cheese, coconut oil, eggs and vinegar and stir everything.
4. Add broccoli and stir again.
5. Shape 12 patties, arrange on a baking sheet, introduce in the oven at 375 degrees F and bake for 20 minutes.
6. Turn the oven to broiler and broil your biscuits for 5 minutes more.
7. Arrange on a platter and serve.

Enjoy!

Nutrition: calories 163, fat 12, fiber 2, carbs 2, protein 7

Tasty Corndogs

These are so delicious and simple to make!

Preparation time: 10 minutes
Cooking time: 10 minutes
Servings: 4

Ingredients:

- 1 and ½ cups olive oil
- 2 tablespoons heavy cream
- 1 cup almond meal
- 4 sausages
- 1 teaspoon baking powder
- 1 teaspoon Italian seasoning
- 2 eggs
- ½ teaspoon turmeric
- Salt and black pepper to the taste
- A pinch of cayenne pepper

Directions:

1. In a bowl, mix almond meal with Italian seasoning, baking powder, turmeric, salt, pepper and cayenne and stir well.

2. In another bowl, mix eggs with heavy cream and whisk well.
3. Combine the 2 mixtures and stir well.
4. Dip sausages in this mix and place them on a plate.
5. Heat up a pan with the oil over medium high heat, add sausages, cook for 2 minutes on each side and transfer to paper towels.
6. Drain grease, arrange on a platter and serve.

Enjoy!

Nutrition: calories 345, fat 33, fiber 4, carbs 5, protein 16

Tasty Pepper Nachos

These look wonderful! They are so tasty and healthy!

Preparation time: 10 minutes
Cooking time: 20 minutes
Servings: 6

Ingredients:

- 1 pound mini bell peppers, cut in halves
- Salt and black pepper to the taste
- 1 teaspoon garlic powder
- 1 teaspoon sweet paprika
- ½ teaspoon oregano, dried
- ¼ teaspoon red pepper flakes
- 1 pound beef meat, ground
- 1 and ½ cups cheddar cheese, shredded
- 1 tablespoons chili powder
- 1 teaspoon cumin, ground
- ½ cup tomato, chopped
- Sour cream for serving

Directions:

1. In a bowl, mix chili powder with paprika, salt, pepper, cumin, oregano, pepper flakes and garlic powder and stir.
2. Heat up a pan over medium heat, add beef, stir and brown for 10 minutes.
3. Add chili powder mix, stir and take off heat.
4. Arrange pepper halves on a lined baking sheet, stuff them with the beef mix, sprinkle cheese, introduce in the oven at 400 degrees F and bake for 10 minutes.
5. Take peppers out of the oven, sprinkle tomatoes and divide between plates and serve with sour cream on top.

Enjoy!

Nutrition: calories 350, fat 22, fiber 3, carbs 6, protein 27

Almond Butter Bars

This is a great keto snack for a casual day!

Preparation time: 2 hours and 10 minutes
Cooking time: 2 minutes
Servings: 12

Ingredients:

- ¾ cup coconut, unsweetened and shredded
- ¾ cup almond butter
- ¾ cup stevia
- 1 cup almond butter
- 2 tablespoons almond butter
- 4.5 ounces dark chocolate, chopped
- 2 tablespoons coconut oil

Directions:

1. In a bowl, mix almond flour with stevia and coconut and stir well.
2. Heat up a pan over medium-low heat, add 1 cup almond butter and the coconut oil and whisk well.
3. Add this to almond flour and stir well.
4. Transfer this to a baking dish and press well.

5. Heat up another pan with the chocolate stirring often.
6. Add the rest of the almond butter and whisk well again.
7. Pour this over almond mix and spread evenly.
8. Introduce in the fridge for 2 hours, cut into 12 bars and serve as a keto snack.

Enjoy!

Nutrition: calories 140, fat 2, fiber 1, carbs 5, protein 1

Conclusion

This is really a life changing cookbook. It shows you everything you need to know about the Ketogenic diet and it helps you get started.
You now know some of the best and most popular Ketogenic recipes in the world.
We have something for everyone's taste!

So, don't hesitate too much and start your new life as a follower of the Ketogenic diet!
Get your hands on this special recipes collection and start cooking in this new, exciting and healthy way!

Have a lot of fun and enjoy your Ketogenic diet!

Lightning Source UK Ltd.
Milton Keynes UK
UKHW020642060521
383241UK00015B/1096